Copyright ©2019, Ketoveo

All rights reserved. No part of this publication may be reproduced, distributed or transmitted in any form or by any means, including photocopying, recording, or other electronic or mechanical methods, without the prior written permission of the publisher, except in the case of brief quotations embodied in critical reviews and certain other noncommercial uses permitted by copyright law.

Although the author and publisher have made every effort to ensure that the information in this book was correct at press time, the author and publisher do not assume and hereby disclaim any liability to any party for any loss, damage, or disruption caused by errors or omissions, whether such errors or omissions result from negligence, accident, or any other cause.

Nutritional values have been calculated with due care and attention. However, there may be differences due to the variance of each individual kitchen creation caused by ingredient amounts, brand differences, different cuts and quality of meats etc. The nutritional values of these recipes are provided as a guideline only.

Disclaimer – this book is not intended to be a substitute for the medical advice of a licensed physician. The reader should consult with their doctor in any matters relating to their health. The information provided within this book is for general informational purposes only. While we try to keep the information up-to-date and correct, there are no representations or warranties, express or implied, about the completeness, accuracy, reliability, suitability, or availability with respect to the information, products, services, or related graphics/pictures contained in this book for any purpose. Any use of this information is at your own risk.

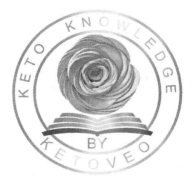

Go to **www.ketoveo.com** for more guides and resources to help you on your keto journey.

CONTENTS

Introduction	1-2
Chapter 1: What is a Ketogenic Diet?	3
Chapter 2: Benefits of the Keto Diet	4
Sugar vs Ketones	5
Keto Diet & Diabetes	6
Keto Diet & Alzheimer's Disease	6
Keto Diet & Fatigue	7
Keto Diet & Acne	8
Keto Diet & Aging	9
Keto Diet & Autism	10
Chapter 3: The ingredients of a Keto Diet	11
Seafood	
Vegetables (low-carb vegetables)	
Diary	
Avocados	
Meat & Poultry	15
Eggs	16
Coconut Oil	16
Dark Chocolate/ Cocoa Powder	17
Chapter 4: Foods to Avoid	18
Processed Foods	18
Boxed Cereals	19
White Flours & White Rice	19
Legumes	20
Alcohol	20
Counting Carbs	21
Chapter 5: Keto Friendly Food	22-27
Shopping List	28-29

Chapter 6: The Keto Diet for Rapid Weight Loss ... 30
Keto vs Low Carb ... 31
Keto vs Paleo ... 32
Keto vs Atkins ... 33
The Ketogenic Diet ... 34
Ketosis Explained ... 35
Keto Symptoms ... 36
Intermittent Fasting on a Keto Diet ... 37
Chapter 7: Let the Keto Journey Begin ... 38
Time to Clean Out the Pantry ... 38
Weigh Yourself ... 39
Get Smart with Substitutes ... 39
Condiments are Not Your Friend ... 40
Watch your Ketones ... 40
What about Eating Out ... 41
Get your Protein & Exercise ... 42
Endgame ... 43
Glossary ... 44-46

WHAT IS KETO?

Introduction

If you are eating a high-carbohydrate diet, you are most likely eating a lot of processed food and high doses of sugar. In doing so, you are not giving your body the nutrients it needs. Instead, you are adding up the calories and potentially increasing your risk of disease. So, what is the solution?

The moment you type the letter 'k' in a Google search, 8 times out of 10, the Ketogenic Diet (or simply Keto Diet) would show up as a search result. What is the Keto Diet? Is it one of those diets which is just an old book with a new cover? Is it an over-blown fad which no one has ever really completed but yet everyone can't stop singing its praises? In a world ruled by buzzwords, is it one of those hyped up diets which one random celebrity came up with and now everyone is doing it?

The answer to all these questions is - no.
First and foremost, the Keto Diet is one of the few diets known which is based on actual solid science. The word 'Keto' is derived from the word ketosis which is the state that the human body goes into where instead of burning carbohydrates (starches and sugars) to generate energy, your body burns stored fat.

Your marvelous human body can use both carbohydrates and fat as the source of energy. But it's inclined to use carbohydrates as the primary source. The main goal of the Keto Diet is to break away from this process and get your body to use fat as its primary fuel.

But how does your body do that?

Well, it needs a little help from you. If you decreased or removed carbohydrates from your diet, your body would have no choice but to shift over to the alternative source. It would begin to consume the stored fat.

But this brings another question, why are carbohydrates the villain here? Let's talk about it first. When you eat high-carb food, it breaks down into glucose before being absorbed into the bloodstream. From this point on, it enters your body cells with the help of insulin. Glucose is used by your body for energy and any unused glucose is converted into glycogen. When more glucose is consumed than that which can be stored as glycogen, it converts to fat. So, now we can see, more carbs means more glucose, more glucose means more fat, and more fat means weight gain.

Imagine, if you had two sources of energy and using one of them causes more harm than good, and then you find out that using the second one will not only provide you enough energy, it will also make you stronger and more fit. This is what the Keto Diet does for your body.

Low-carb intake drives your body to go into the state of ketosis. During ketosis your body is trained to use fat as the main source of energy instead of carbs. Your liver plays an important role in ketosis. When it realizes that there is not enough fuel in the form of carbs to power your body, it breaks down fat into ketones, which in turn allows your body to use fat as energy. You don't stop eating food, you just stop eating carbohydrate-rich food. This process, in tandem with a good workout routine, makes weight loss a walk in the park. And it just doesn't stop at weight loss, it helps you control and fight a lot of other diseases as well.

As with all things that provide great results, "going Keto" comes with an equal amount of hard work. For someone with a sweet-tooth, it is indeed going to be tricky to avoid sugar. But as the saying goes "If it was easy, everyone would have done it." In the end, you'll realize that it was worth the price because you'll feel more fit both physically and mentally.

Chapter 1

What is a Ketogenic Diet?

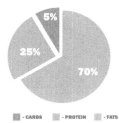

The Ketogenic Diet is the process of manipulating your body to switch its energy source from carbohydrates to the fat which has been stored in your body or which you eat. You do this by controlling the ratio of carbs, fats, and proteins which you consume.

As mentioned earlier, excess fat is the reason we keep adding pounds. In a typical diet, the focus is on working out and then keeping a close eye on the number of calories being consumed. On top of that, you need to make sure that the quantity of calories you burn is always greater than the calorie intake. Because so many variables are involved, it gets difficult which is why people stop following their diet and go back to gaining weight.

A Ketogenic Diet is not only about weight loss. It also helps to control the glucose, or blood sugar in your body. Too much sugar in your body forces the pancreas to work harder to pump out more insulin.

As with any machine, if you keep pushing it to the limit, there comes a point when it will break or stop working at its maximum efficiency. Without enough insulin, the sugar concentration in the blood keeps getting higher and higher and leads to the disease called diabetes. And with diabetes comes high blood pressure, heart disease, kidney disease, and many other maladies.

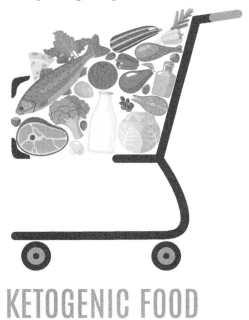

In the Ketogenic Diet we simply need to keep in mind that this is a low-carb, moderate protein, and high fat diet. Compose your daily meals to be 5% carbs, 25% proteins and 70% Fat.

The crucial manipulation of carbs, fats, and protein in a Ketogenic Diet leads to ketosis and you know the rest of the story now.
To state it simply, a Ketogenic Diet can help you lose much more weight than a low-fat diet and it does it without making you super hungry.

Chapter 2

Benefits of the Keto Diet

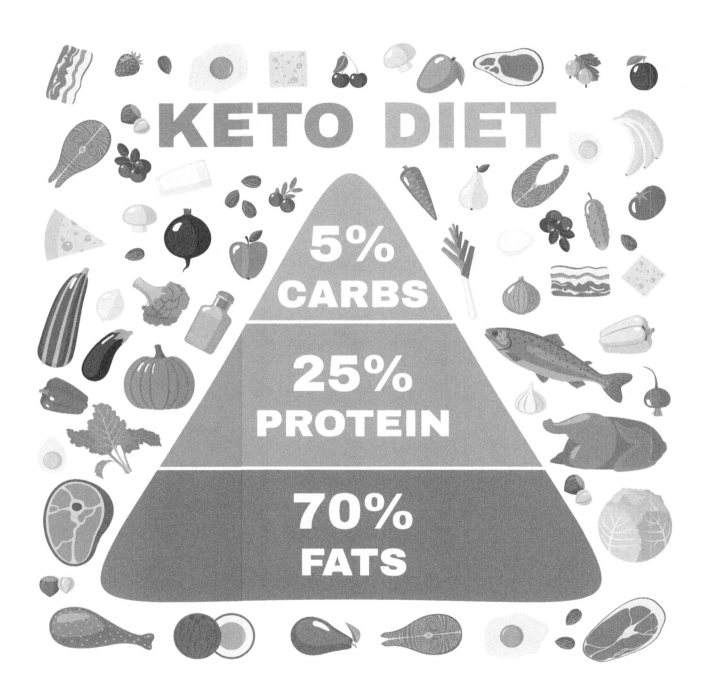

Sugar vs Ketones

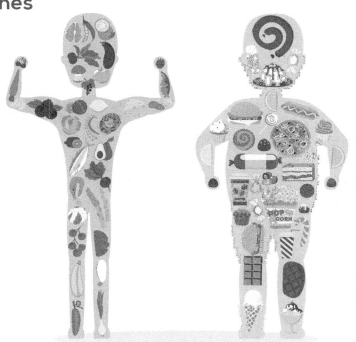

So far, what we are sure of is that the Keto Diet is basically the replacement of carbs by fats as the main source of energy. This, as mentioned before, is the condition called ketosis. The actual fuel being used during ketosis is called ketones. These ketones and sugar do basically the same thing, but how they affect your body cannot be more different. Let's compare the two.

When you eat food, you increase the number of free radicals in your body. Free radicals are types of oxygen-containing molecules which strongly interact with other molecules. But not in a good way. These reactions cause damage to your cells, protein and DNA.

Usually, these free radicals are kept in check by antioxidants. Your body makes some of the antioxidants it needs and some you get from the food you eat. In theory, you have enough antioxidants operating and your body keeps on its merry way to stay healthy. But with an excessive consumption of sugar/carbs, you get too many free radicals and your body's ability to produce enough antioxidants falls far behind and these free radicals then start damaging your organs and functions of your body .

Additionally, a high intake of simple sugars can make cells, including your brain cells, insulin resistant which could cause brain cells to die. On the other hand, ketones help protect the cells in your body by reducing the production of free radicals in your body . This, in turn, has shown to protect neuron cells in the brain. The healthy cells of your body which are being affected by high doses of sugar are also helped by these ketones. It is done by improving the cell health and protecting it from damaging inflammation.

One thing we all need to understand is that there is more to the Ketogenic Diet than just a rapid weight loss technique. It comes with important medical benefits.

Keto Diet & Diabetes

We have established that by utilizing the Ketogenic Diet, you are able to control the amount of glucose in your blood which will then help you to avoid diabetes or at least to control it. Also, Anyone who knows anything about diabetes would tell you that one of the biggest risks is cataracts. Here again, a Keto Diet could help. With active control over carbs and sugar, it could fight to keep any eye related issues at bay and enjoy better vision.

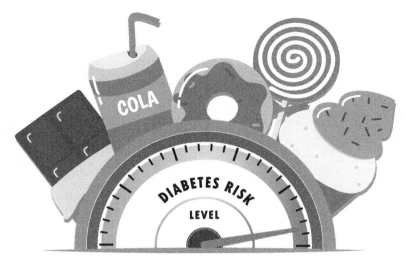

In a recent study, clear signs were found that people with type 2 diabetes are twice as likely to have Alzheimer's than someone who is not a diabetic.

Keto Diet & Alzheimer's Disease

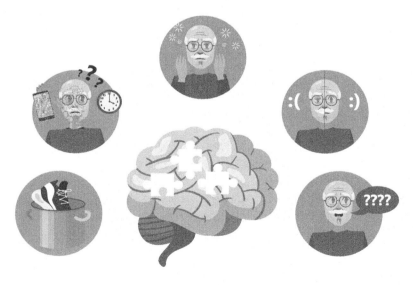

Another study done in 2012 showed that people who ate a high-carb diet had an 80% higher chance of developing mild cognitive impairment. Or in other words, they are on the road to dementia. Although genetic and non-nutritional factors are also responsible for Alzheimer's, more and more people are realizing that food is one factor that can be controlled, and the Ketogenic Diet seems like the be the first step forward.

Since the Ketogenic Diet leads to a healthier and enhanced brain function, it's a wise choice for those seeking a better and healthier brain.

Keto Diet & Fatigue

Do you feel tired on a regular basis? Maybe it's time to look at your diet. If you are on a high-carbohydrate diet, you will feel tired easily. The reason behind this is that carbs are not an efficient source of energy when compared to fats. If you need more efficiency from your body's engine, then you must feed it high-efficiency fuel which (as you must have correctly guessed by now) is fat.

Thus, a Ketogenic Diet can surely put you on the path to becoming the Energizer Bunny of human beings. When you have a more efficient power source, you have a higher output. This holds true for machines as well as humans.

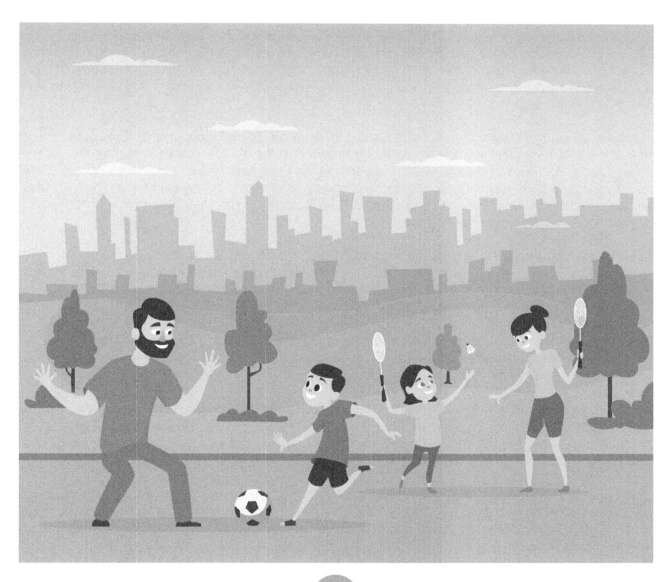

Keto Diet & Acne

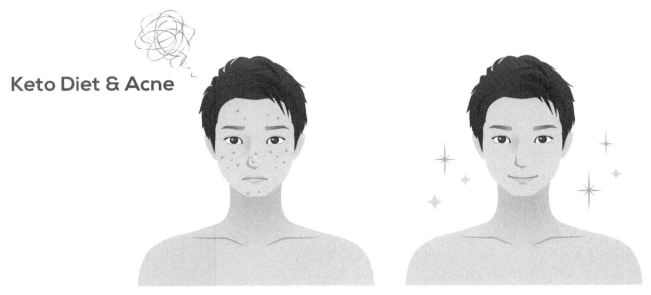

Every time you turn on the TV, you can almost bet that in the first ad break, there will most likely be an ad about acne. You must be wondering why are we talking about acne in a Keto book. Let's dive deeper and see how our favorite villain - carbohydrates - is related to acne and how the Keto Diet can fight that problem.

IGF-1 is a hormone produced by your pituitary gland whose task is to tell your body how many cells to create. Also known as a growth hormone, it controls the rate of creation of new cells and the replacement of the older ones. Under normal circumstances, IGF-1 is needed and does its job well.

However, when the levels of IGF-1 start going over normal, it triggers the creation of a lot of new skin cells. Even though these cells are created beneath the surface of the skin, they slowly rise, and you can guess what happens when they reach the top. There are already cells there and thus begins competition for space and resources. As a result, they end up blocking the pores and they provide the optimal condition for infection, inflammation and the teenager's greatest enemy: acne.

It doesn't stop there. Increased IGF-1 levels mean more sebum. Sebum is an oil naturally produced by your body to keep your skin moisturized and to protect it against bacteria. But excess sebum can lead to blocked pores which in turn leads to acne. So excess IFG-1 starts a chain reaction which can lead to acne.

This brings up the question, what could cause excess IGF-1 to be produced? The answer is: carbohydrates. If you have been eating a high-carb diet and are wondering why you have acne, now you know who the culprit is here.

On the other side is the Ketogenic Diet, where you control the intake of carbohydrates, which implies less glucose and sugar in your body and this, in turn, keeps IFG-1 levels from overflowing. Once this overflow is avoided, the conditions are ripe for you to have an acne free face.

Having too many carbs in your diet is definitely one of the reasons which can cause acne, however, there are others. But the food you eat is something that is completely in your control and if you decide to follow the Ketogenic Diet way, you have a good shot at having clearer, healthier skin

Keto Diet & Aging

That brings us to the next benefit: the Ketogenic Diet is anti-aging. How? Let's look at the information we have gathered so far.

We all start our human journey from one cell. This cell divides into two and then these two cells split into four and so on and so forth. All these cells combine to form different parts of our body. But there is a limit to how many times each cell can divide, and this limit is called the Hayflick limit. One cell divides approximately fifty times and then it reaches the Hayflick limit, stops dividing and begins to die.

Now think of what we have learned and found earlier in this article: the Ketogenic Diet enhances the health of our cells while sugar degrades them. With the Ketogenic Diet, our cells stay healthy longer and perform better, which in turn means the average lifetime of a cell increases and thus our body is able to stay "younger" for longer which delays the natural aging process.

The Ketogenic Diet enhances the ability of the little power plants in our bodies, called mitochondria, to provide energy in a manner that reduces inflammation and oxidative stress. Although the studies on this have been limited, it makes sense to assume that this diet can help us feeling and looking younger and stronger for longer than the sugar-rich carbohydrate diets that the average person consumes every day.

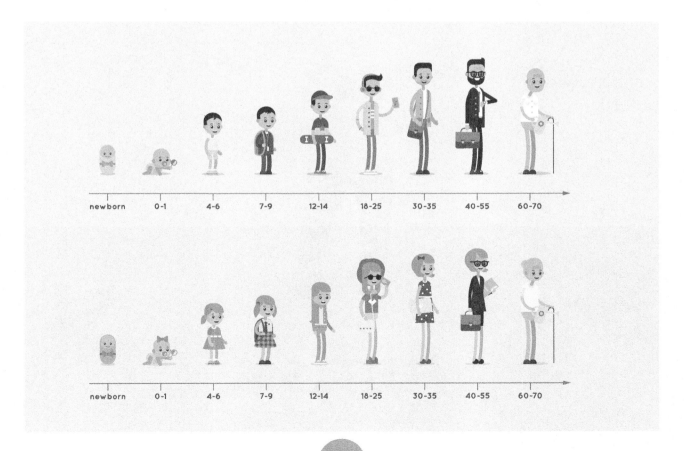

Keto Diet & Autism

In 2018, a study was published which showed a significant reduction in symptoms for some autistic children on the Ketogenic Diet. It is known that inflammation is an important factor in causing autism. Since the Ketogenic Diet can help control inflammation, it is an effective asset dealing with autistic symptoms.

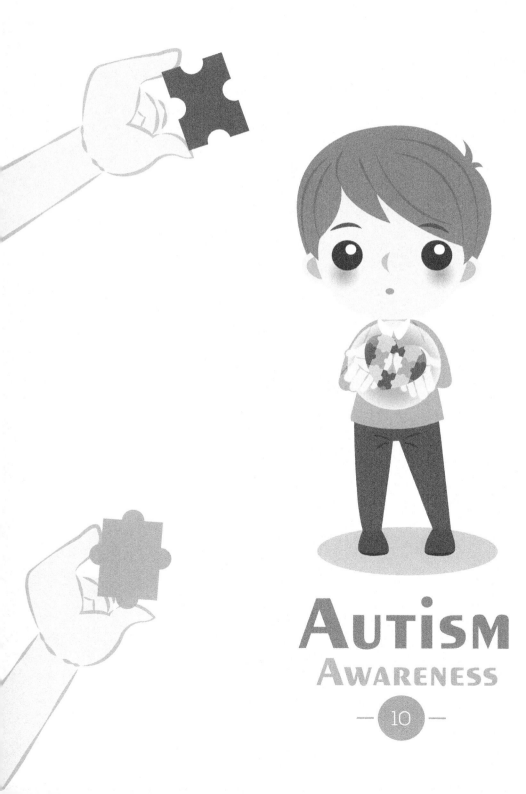

Chapter 3

The Ingredients of a Keto Diet

Most people do not associate fats with being healthy and strong. But after an introduction to the Ketogenic Diet, maybe it's time we stopped looking at fats as an enemy but instead saw them as an ally in our battle against unhealthy living. Let's look at some examples and figure out what exactly a Ketogenic Diet is composed of.

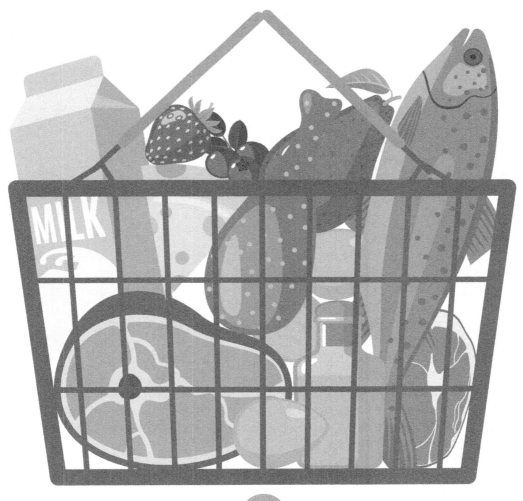

SEAFOOD

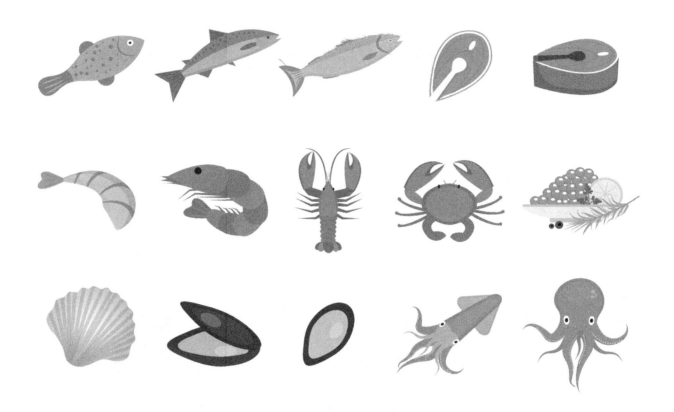

Fish are often called "brain food" because they can provide the necessary nutrition to the brain cells due to the omega-3 and omega-6 fatty acids found in them. The human brain is nearly 60 percent fat. Fatty acids are among the most crucial components that determine your brain's integrity and ability to perform. Since brain tissue primarily consists of fatty acids, any diet that provides these will likely improve your brain.

Salmon and other fish should be one of your main foods. Fish is also high in vitamins and minerals. Best of all, they are virtually carb-free. But keep an eye on the carb content of shellfish. Salmon can easily be the king of the Ketogenic Diet as it not only consists of almost no carbs, it is also very high in omega-3 fatty acids and has been shown to lower insulin levels. It is also known to increase insulin sensitivity in overweight and obese young adults. Eating twice per week should be your target.

VEGETABLES (low-carb vegetables)

If it's green and leafy, gobble it up as soon as you can. It's the best advice you can give to anyone. Many vegetables are very low-carb and filled with almost every possible vitamin and mineral known to mankind.

They have the added advantage that they are full of fiber. Although fiber is technically a carbohydrate, your body cannot fully digest it and therefore it cannot be broken down into sugar molecules. Fiber is great for helping regulate blood sugar and hunger.

Remember the free-radicals we spoke about earlier? Vegetables contain antioxidants which can help protect against free radicals and prevent cell damage. Spinach, brussels sprouts, kale, broccoli, and cauliflower are the best replacements for any high-carb diet.

But not all vegetables will work on a Keto Diet. You will want to steer away from potatoes, yams, corn and other high-starch vegetables as they will turn the tables on your diet very easily and quickly.

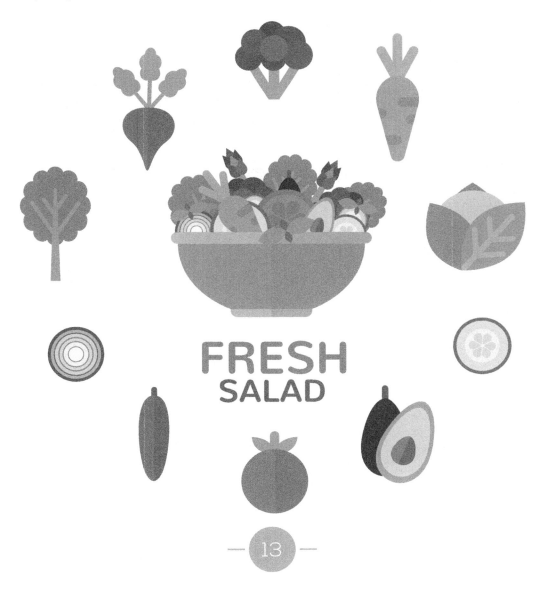

DAIRY

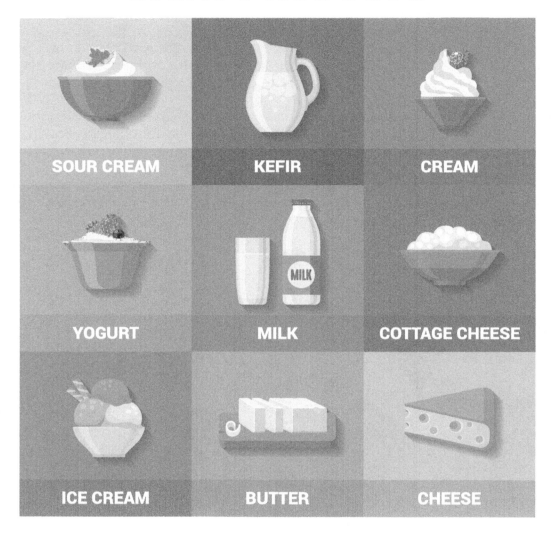

Cheese is something that will not only add to the taste of your Keto Diet, it is also something that will give you a high amount of fat, protein, and calcium.

Yogurt is a wonderful source of protein and calcium. Plain Greek yogurt may have no fat in it, but it has only 7 grams of carbs and a whopping 24 grams of protein in a cup. But remember to stay away from the flavored ones, they will upturn your Keto cart in one meal. They are a storehouse for sugar. If you want a bit of flavor, add a few berries to the yogurt to satisfy your taste buds.

AVOCADOS

Avocados are the numero uno of the Keto Diet. It is 15% fat, most of which is the type of fat which helps to lower bad cholesterol. As well, avocados have loads of vitamins and minerals. No wonder it is called a superfood.

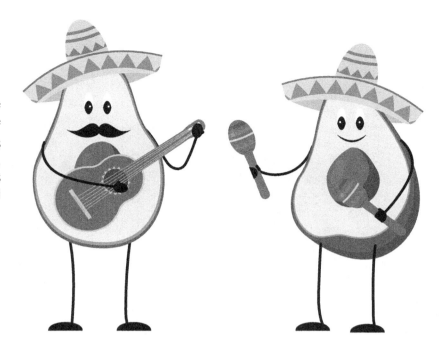

MEAT & POULTRY

Meat and poultry are staples of the Keto Diet. Low on carbs and high on proteins and fat, they can fit into just about any meal. A study that was done on Australian beef found animals that are grass fed produce meat with higher amounts of omega-3 and antioxidants than meat from grain fed animals. Whether it is the chicken thighs or the New York strip steak, they will keep your fat and protein intake in sync with your Keto plan.

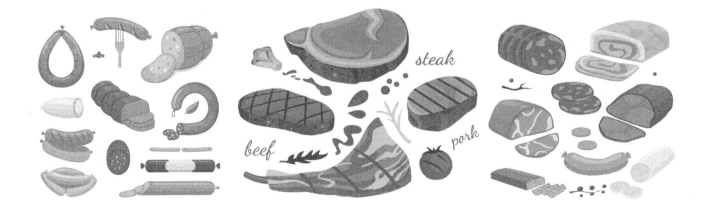

EGGS

Eggs truly are incredible. They are high in protein, high in fat, and very low on carbs. A boiled egg contains around 11 grams of fat, 13 grams of protein, and only 1 gram of carbs. Eggs are one of the most nutrient dense foods on the planet! For most people, eating the yolk doesn't increase the cholesterol in your body very much, but if one is diabetic, it might be best to stay away from the yolk and stick to the egg whites.

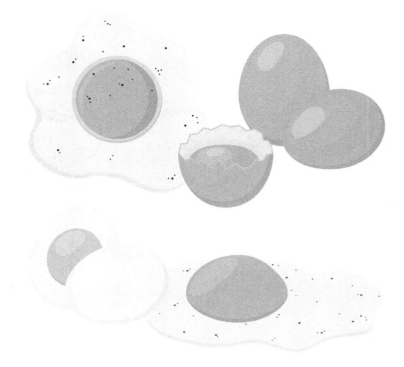

COCONUT OIL

MCT (Medium-chain triglycerides) are found in coconuts and can aid in weight loss. Their specialty is that (unlike the long-chain triglycerides) they metabolize differently and go directly to the liver, where they are turned into ketones.

These ketones are what we need for a successful Ketogenic Diet. These ketones can cross from the blood to the brain and can provide an alternate source of energy for the brain. Moreover, since the calories contained in the MCTs are burnt more efficiently and used by your body, the probability of them being stored as fat is minimal.

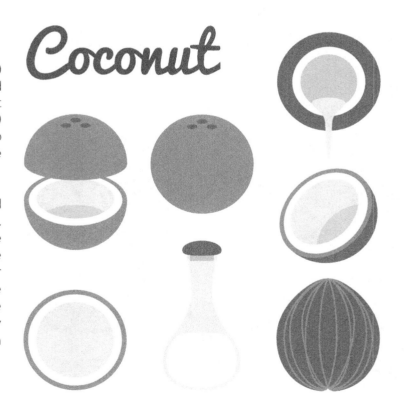

DARK CHOCOLATE/ COCOA POWDER

Considered one of the best sources of antioxidants on the planet, a 70-85% dark chocolate is a great option for dessert on the Keto Diet. Just make sure the chocolate you enjoy is sugar-free. Luckily there are many chocolate bars made today using Erythritol, Stevia or other non-sugar sweeteners.

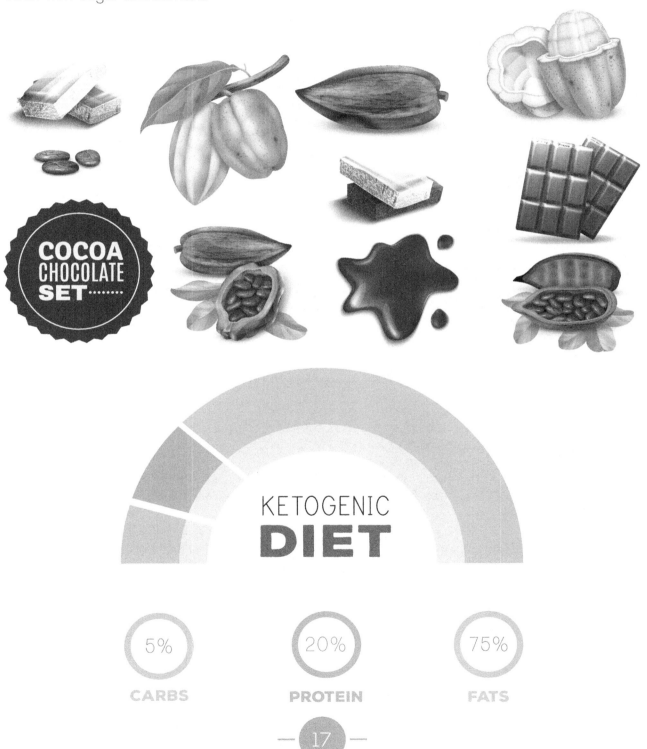

Chapter 4

Foods to Avoid

Every diet plan has two major parts to it: things you can eat and things you cannot eat. We have spoken at length about the things you can eat, why they are important and how they help. Now it's time to look on the flip side - things not to eat and why you should not be eating them.

PROCESSED FOODS

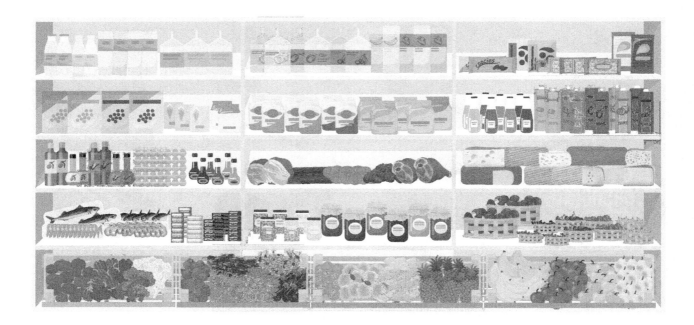

The top of this list is any type of processed food. They are carbohydrate headquarters and should be skipped altogether during your grocery runs.

Mother Nature has all the foods that we require, and the healthiest option is to use it all naturally. Processed foods are filled with preservatives and chemicals. These need to be avoided at all costs.

A good idea is to make a habit of reading the Nutritional Facts labels on foods. A word of caution here, even food labels have an uncanny ability to "hide" important information. Often you can look at a label and see "Sugars 0g", and feel that it's something worth buying. But when you look a couple of lines above that you will see "Total Carbohydrate" which could well be in double digits. A rule of thumb is to not focus on the one-line item when looking at a label. Read the whole thing and then decide.

BOXED CEREALS

Keep your guard up when it comes to boxed cereals. Most popular brands are pretty much devoid of anything which can nourish your body. The box will say a lot of fancy things on it, but one look at the label and you will know that it's something to stay away from. Unless you can find something that is natural with a high amount of fiber and low or no carbs in it, it is best to stay away.

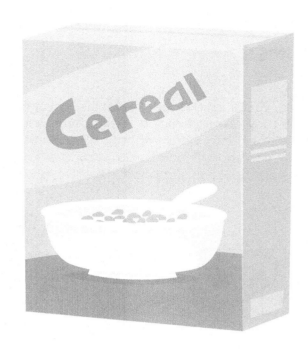

WHITE FLOURS & WHITE RICE

White bread, pasta, and white rice have been stripped of the majority of nutrients and are full of starch. And starches are pure carbohydrate. You can guess what starch leads to: a glucose filled trip which will affect every possible body part in a negative way. So stay away from white bread and its comrades.

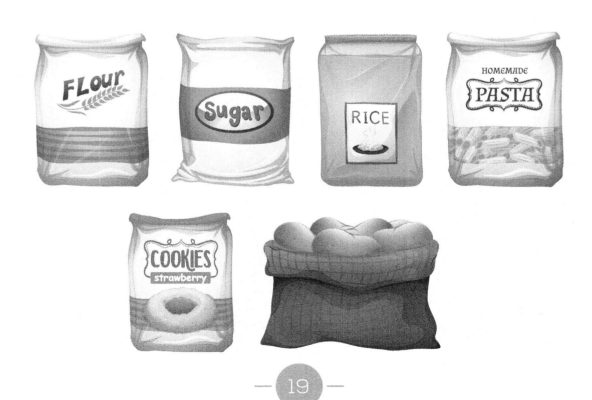

LEGUMES

Legumes, which include beans, lentils, peas and peanuts, seem like they would be an ally because they are so full of protein. Unfortunately, they are also full of carbs. For example, 100 grams of kidney beans contains 24 grams of protein but they also contain 35 grams of the carbs you should avoid. Since legumes do provide a lot of protein, it may be a good idea to keep your daily consumption in the 20-50 gram count. (see Counting Carbs below).

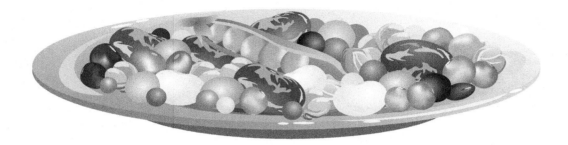

ALCOHOL

Alcohol is a tricky one. Beer should not be on your drinking list as just one beer will take up a large chunk of your carb limit for the day. Pure alcohols, such as whiskey, vodka, brandy, gin and tequila have no fats or carbs. When you drink alcohol, the first organ that gets affected negatively is your liver. When your liver tries to break down alcohol, it damages its cells. You need to protect your liver, especially in a Ketogenic Diet because this is where all your precious ketones are made.

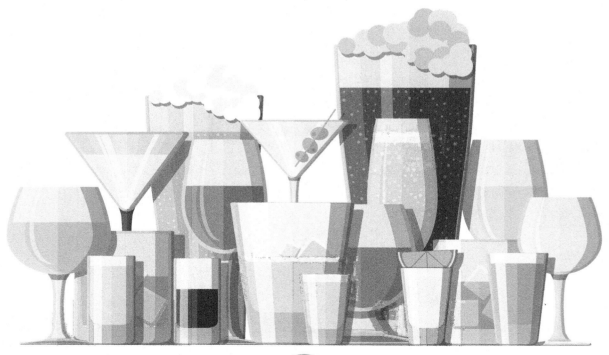

COUNTING CARBS

An important factor to understand is knowing how to choose the carbs that are OK and which you should avoid. What you want to consider when determining the quantity of carbs is to pay most attention to "net carbs". To determine the net carbs of most any food, look at the Nutritional Facts table on the foods you buy.

Use this formula:

Total Carbohydrate minus Dietary Fiber equals Net Carbs. For example, in a typical avocado, there are a total of twelve grams of carbohydrate. However, subtract the ten grams of dietary fiber and the net carbs is only two. This is less than 1.5% of the whole avocado. On the other hand, a typical apple has 25 grams of total carbohydrate of which only 4 are dietary fiber. Net carbs of an apple are 20 grams which is 21% of the whole apple. A huge difference!

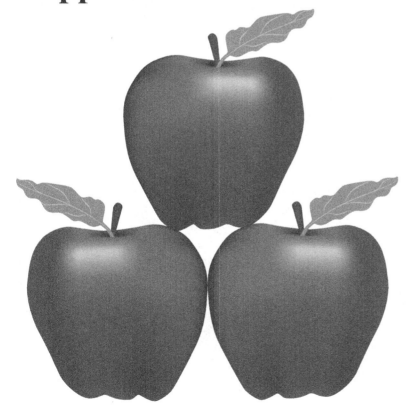

Apple Nutrition Facts

Nutrition Facts	
Serving Size 1 Apple (medium) 132 g	
Amount Per Serving	
Calories 95	Calories from fat 3
	% Daily Value*
Total Fat 0g	0%
Saturated Fat 0g	0%
Trans Fat 0g	
Cholesterol 0g	0%
Sodium 2mg	0%
Total Carbohydrate 25g	8%
Dietary Fiber 4g	17%
Sugars 19g	
Protein 0g	
Vitamin A	2%
Vitamin C	14%
Calcium	1%
Iron	1%
*Percent Daily Values are based on a 2,000 calorie diet. Your daily values may be higher or lower depending on your calorie needs.	

Keto Friendly Food

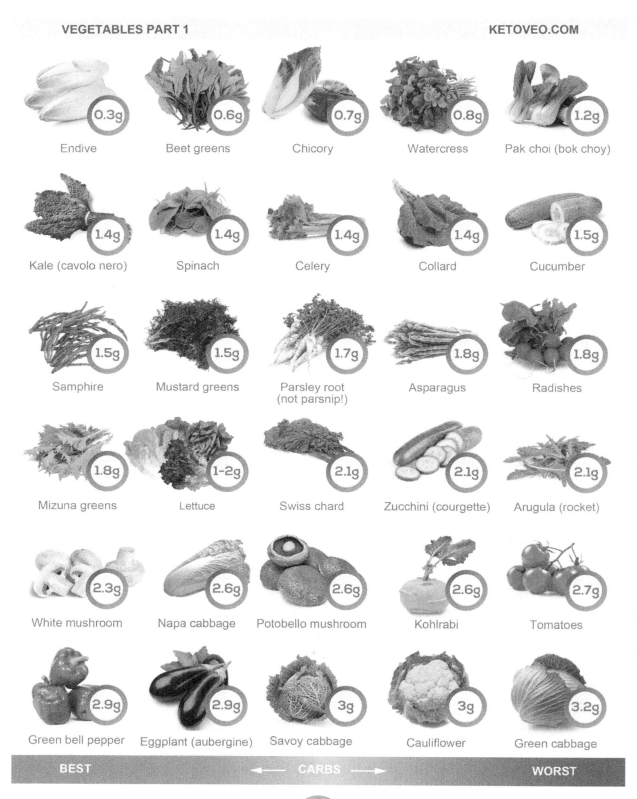

VEGETABLES PART 2

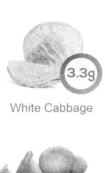 White Cabbage — 3.3g
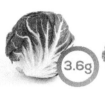 Radicchio — 3.6g
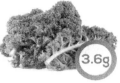 Kale (curly) — 3.6g
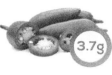 Jalapeno peppers — 3.7g
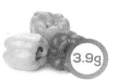 Other bell pepper — 3.9g

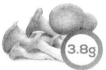 Oyster mushroom — 3.8g
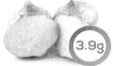 Jicama — 3.9g
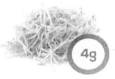 Bean sprouts — 4g
Broccoli — 4g
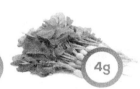 Daikon radish — 4g

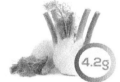 Fennel — 4.2g
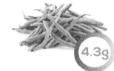 Green beans — 4.3g
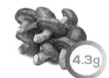 Shiitake mushroom — 4.3g
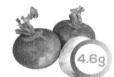 Turnip — 4.6g
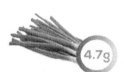 Spring Onion — 4.7g

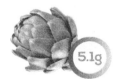 Artichoke (globe) — 5.1g
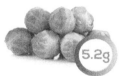 Brussel sprouts — 5.2g
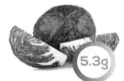 Red cabbage — 5.3g
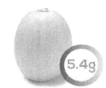 Spaghetti squash — 5.4g
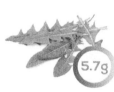 Dandelion greens — 5.7g

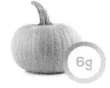 Pie pumpkin — 6g
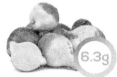 Rutabaga (swede) — 6.3g
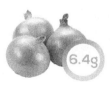 Brown onion — 6.4g
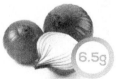 Red onion — 6.5g
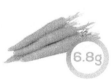 Carrot — 6.8g

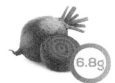 Beetroot — 6.8g
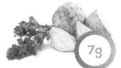 Celeriac — 7g
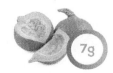 Hokkaido squash — 7g
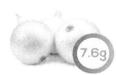 White onion — 7.6g
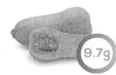 Butter squash — 9.7g

BEST ← CARBS → **WORST**

DRINKS

KETOVEO.COM

Drink	Carbs	Serving
Water with lemon	0	1 cup
Tea	0	1 cup
Coffee	0	1 cup
Coconut water	9	1 cup
Vegetable juice	11*	1 cup
Milk	11*	1 cup
Soy milk	12*	1 cup
Caffè latte	15	12 oz
Orange juice	26	1 cup
Energy drink	28	8,4 oz
Ice tea	32	12 oz
Smoothie	36	1 cup
Soft drink	39	12 oz
Frappuccino	50	12 oz
Milkshake	60	10 oz

BEST ← CARBS → WORST

CONDIMENTS AND MORE

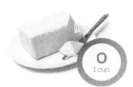
Butter — 0 (1 cup)

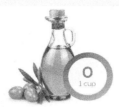
Olive oil — 0 (1 cup)

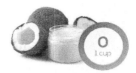
Coconut oil — 0 (1 cup)

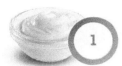
Mayonnaise — 1

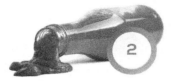
Tabasco / Hot sause — 2

Heavy cream — 3

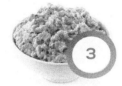
Guacamole — 3

Vinaigrette — 3

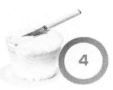
Cream cheese — 4

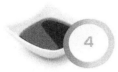
Soy sause — 4

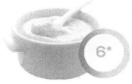
Mustard — 6*

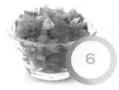
Salsa — 6

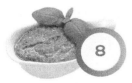
Pesto — 8

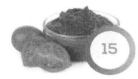
Tomato paste — 15

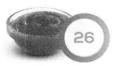
Ketchup — 26

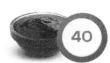
BBQ sause — 40

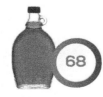
Maple syrup — 68

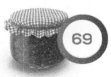
Jam — 69

BEST ← CARBS → WORST

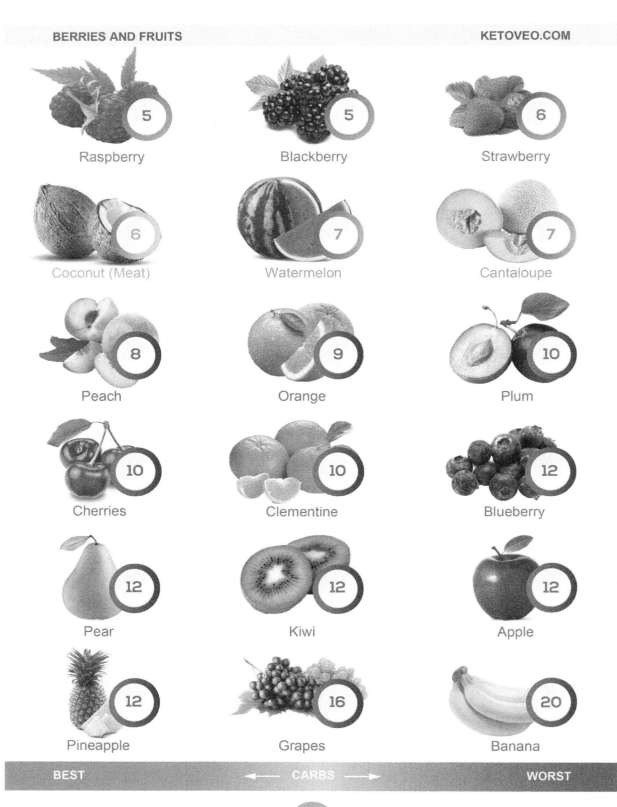

NUTS AND SEEDS

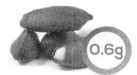 Pili nuts — 0.6g

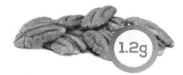 Pecan — 1.2g

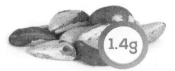 Brazil nuts — 1.4g

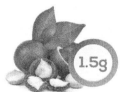 Macadamia — 1.5g

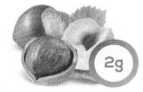 Hazelnut — 2g

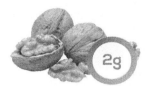 Walnut — 2g

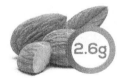 Almonds — 2.6g

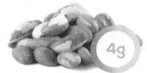 Brazil — 4g

 Pistachio — 5g

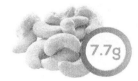 Cashews — 7.7g

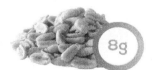 Peanut — 8g

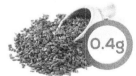 Flax seeds — 0.4g

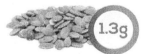 Pumpkin seeds — 1.3g

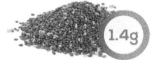 Chia seeds — 1.4g

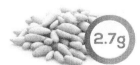 Pine seeds — 2.7g

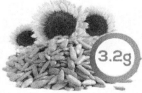 Sunflower seeds — 3.2g

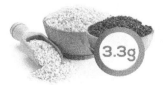 Sesame seeds — 3.3g

BEST ← CARBS → WORST

SHOPPING LIST

BEEF	POULTRY	PORK	SEAFOOD	
• Steak • Prime Rib • Veal • Roast Beef • Brisket • Loin • Ground beef • Stew meats • Organs	• Chicken • Quail • Turkey • Organs • Eggs	• Bacon • Ground pork • Sausage • Bratwurst • Pork rinds • Ham • Pork chops	• Salmon • Tuna • Trout • Cod • Sardines • Tilapia • Shrimp	• Lobster • Crab • Bass • Scallops • Mussels • Clams • Oysters

OTHER • Deli meats • Jerky sticks • Biltong • Salami • Goat • Lamb

LEAFY GREENS		CRUCIFEROUS VEGGIES	
• Spinach • Kale • Swiss chard • Lettuce	• Bok choy • Watercress • Endive • Dandelion greens	• Broccoli • Cauliflower • Red cabbage	• Green cabbage • Napa cabbage • Brussels sprouts

ALL OTHER VEGETABLES AND GREENS

- Avocado
- Asparagus
- Celery
- Spring onion
- Fennel
- Radish
- Kohlrabi
- Jalapeño peppers
- Zucchini
- Eggplant
- Green peppers
- Other bell peppers
- Cucumbers
- Tomatoes
- Spaghetti squash
- Sauerkraut
- White mushrooms
- Portobello mushrooms
- Beetroot
- Brown onion
- Red onion
- Carrots
- Bean sprouts
- Artichoke
- Ginger
- Garlic
- Olives
- Basil
- Sage
- Parsley
- Chives
- Dill

FRUITS AND BERRIES

- Raspberries
- Blackberries
- Strawberries
- Coconut
- Lemon
- Lime
- Starfruit

FATS AND OILS

- Coconut oil
- Olive oil
- Avocado oil
- MCT oil
- Grass fed butter

DAIRY

- Greek yogurt
- Kefir
- Heavy cream
- Half n' Half
- Feta
- Mozzarella
- Cheddar
- Blue cheese
- Parmesan
- Cottage cheese
- Swiss cheese
- Gouda
- Cream cheese
- Colby
- Ricotta
- Brie
- Goat cheese
- Sour cream

DRINKS

- Spring water
- Sparkling water
- Tea
- Coffee
- Bone broth
- Keto greens
- MCT powder mix
- Coconut milk
- Almond milk

CONDIMENTS AND SAUCES

- Apple cider vinegar
- Balsamic vinegar
- Mustard
- Ketchup (sugar free)
- Avocado Mayonnaise
- Salsa
- Lemon juice
- Horseradish
- Lime juice
- Hot sauces
- Soy sauce
- Tabasco

HERBS AND SPICES

- Apple cider vinegar
- Himalayan pink salt
- Sea salt
- Black pepper
- Cilantro
- Cinnamon
- Turmeric
- Cayenne
- Cumin
- Basil
- Thyme
- Sage
- Oregano
- Dill
- Rosemary
- Chili powder
- Paprika

SWEETNERS

- Monk Fruit
- Xylitol
- Lakanto
- Swerve
- Erythritol
- Stevia
- Pyure
- Truvia

CHOCOLATE

- Cocoa Powder
- Cacoa Powder
- Sugar Free Cooking Chocolate
- Dark Chocolate

FLOURS

- Almond Meal
- Almond Flour
- Coconut flour
- Ground Hazelnut flour
- Ground Macadamia flour
- Ground Peanut flour
- Ground Chai Seeds
- Flaxseed Meal
- Sunflower seed meal

THICKENING AGENTS

- Oat Fiber
- Psyllium Husks
- Gelatin
- Glucomannan
- Collagen Protein Powder
- Inulin
- Xanthan gum

Chapter 6

The Keto Diet for Rapid Weight Loss

If you tell anyone that you are working towards weight loss, their response often is something like: "You need to go on a low-carb diet." But you need to understand, it's not that simple and there are many significant differences between a Keto Diet and a low-carb diet.

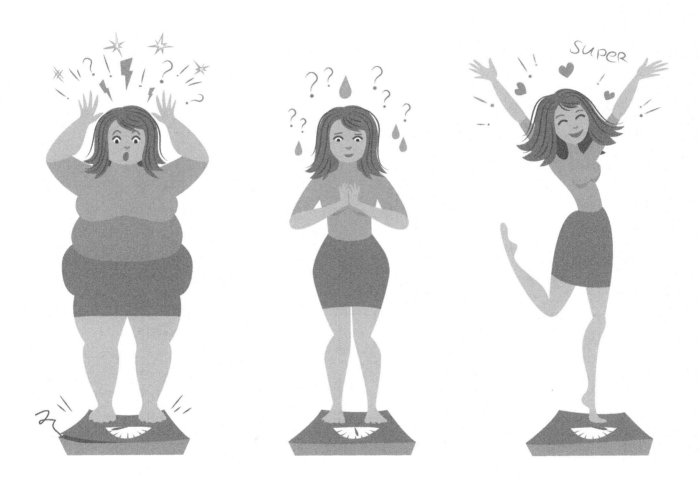

Keto vs Low Carb

If you ask anyone what the definition is of 'low' as in a low-carb diet, you may not get an exact answer. A lot of times, counting carbs can lead to seemingly random choices when looking only at the carb content of a food and deciding whether it should be on your diet or not.

Since there is no defined limit, you may still be eating a lot of carbs and not know it. If you take away carbs from your body and do not replenish it with an alternative source, it will not make you healthy. It will make you hungry, which in turn will make you eat more. On the other hand, Keto has defined limits associated with it and it provides an alternate fuel for your body by using fats.

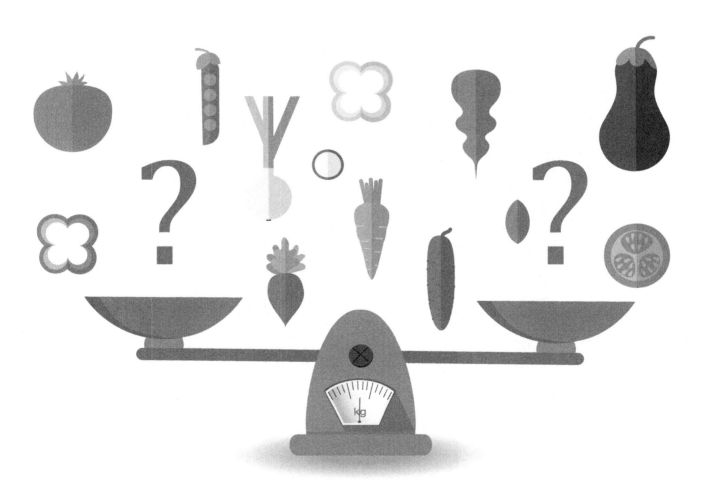

Keto vs Paleo

Many many thousands of years ago when people lived in caves, the diet used to be anything that could be gathered or hunted. The Paleo diet is designed to shift people back onto the same diet. The Paleo Diet focuses on lean meats, fish, fruits, vegetables, nuts, and seeds. The core idea behind Paleo is that the human body is not meant for the modern diet. According to the theory, the new changes in diet brought about by the advent of farming have outpaced your body's ability to adapt.

However, the drawback with Paleo is that there is generally no controlling or manipulating of carbs, proteins, and fats. Therefore, it is at the opposite end of the spectrum when compared to the Keto Diet. Keto is supposed to not only help with weight loss but it is also supposed to be a "healing diet" where it heals the cells and your body .

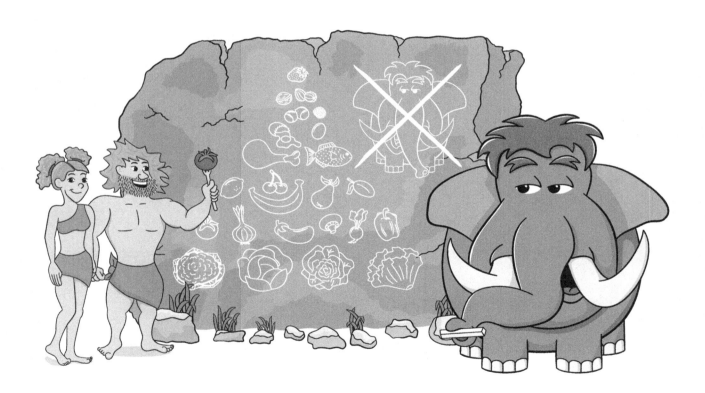

Keto vs Atkins

There are certainly similarities between the Atkins Diet and the Keto Diet. Both are low-carb, hi-fat diets. But with Atkins, you consume low-carb meals only temporarily whereas in Keto, you continue the diet without changing its basic structure in order to maintain your ideal health and weight. By survey, people often have fewer cravings and eat less calories on the Keto Diet.

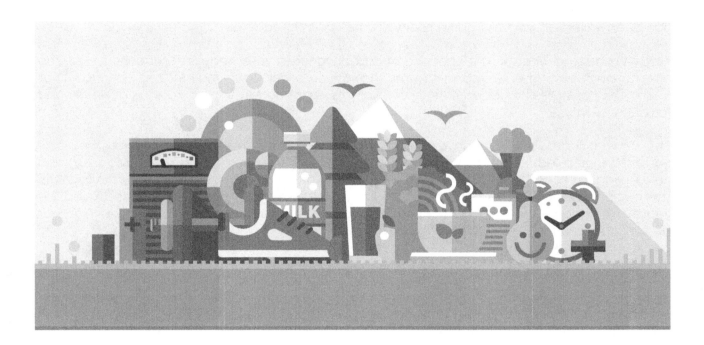

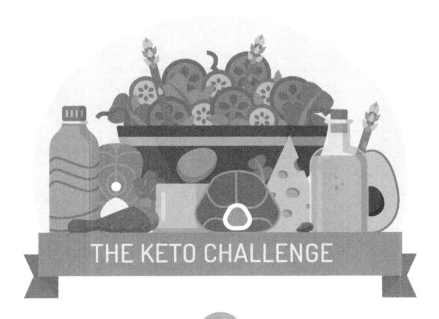

The Ketogenic Diet

Low carbs are only one aspect of the Keto Diet. It not only leads you on your way to losing weight, but it also takes your body to an enhanced state of health and well-being. You feel stronger and more energized, which means no unhealthy snacks can sneak up on you when you have hunger pangs. You control your eating, but you are eating better and healthier.

It's for these reasons that so many people around the world are embracing this amazing diet. It's scientific underpinnings ensure that it works. Ketogenic is not a term coined by some new-age guru, it is a scientifically proven process with nearly a hundred years of history that has been validated and tested by many studies and researches.

Ketosis is a state when, in the absence of carbohydrates, your body is compelled to use the alternative source of energy and it burns the fats stored in your body for this purpose. That is why the Keto Diet has been so successful. This is not something new, it has been around for ages.

The ancient Indian physicians used to fast for days, which led to ketosis which they saw enriched their minds and bodies. Since the early 1920s, the Keto Diet was used to treat and help epileptic children. The Keto Diet is a process which, like any other process, is difficult in the beginning because you are trying to break habits which have been formed over the years. But once you go through the process, you see a healthier and stronger you. Another feature that makes Keto stand out is that there is no deprivation or hunger involved. You do not stop eating, you choose to eat in a better and healthier way.

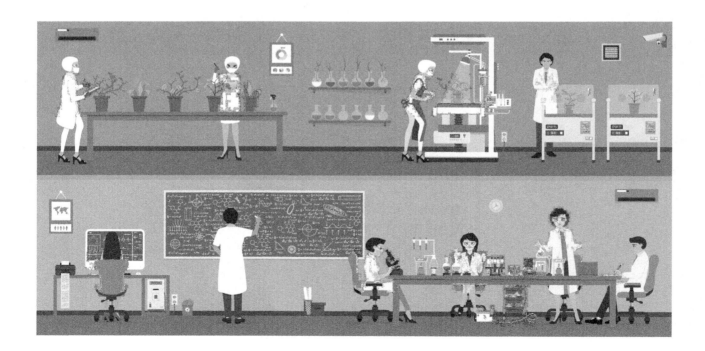

Ketosis Explained

Ketosis is not a spell conjured by Harry Potter. It's a natural occurrence where your body looks for a different pathway to an energy source when it's deprived of its usual path.

At some point in our lives, we have all experienced ketosis, maybe after a strenuous exercise session or when mom forgot to leave lunch in the fridge and we are too lazy to make anything ourselves and therefore your body has started producing ketones to keep us working. Unfortunately, many people eat too much sugar and carbs which prevents ketosis from happening.

A pack of cigarettes has all the warnings on it, yet a smoker ignores all of them. Similarly, we all know the negative effects of excessive sugar and carbs on our bodies, yet we devour them daily. And as a result, we face health issues not limited to weight gain such as diabetes, fatigue, acne, heart disease and so on.

The more you control your intake of carbs, the more your body can produce ketones. Under normal circumstances, fats are stored as an emergency reserve by your body , but during ketosis, it becomes the main source of fuel and you can control it by what you eat and how you eat it.

The Ketogenic Diet is not just a process you follow for a few days and then revert to a diet full of carbs. It is a lifestyle because, as we have mentioned before, so many times it has benefits that go beyond a few pounds off your belly.

Before starting a Keto Diet, you need to first create your goals. Do you simply want to lose weight or are you concerned about your overall health? Is a disease showing its early signs? Always remember, a Keto Diet can be adjusted to suit your needs and goals.

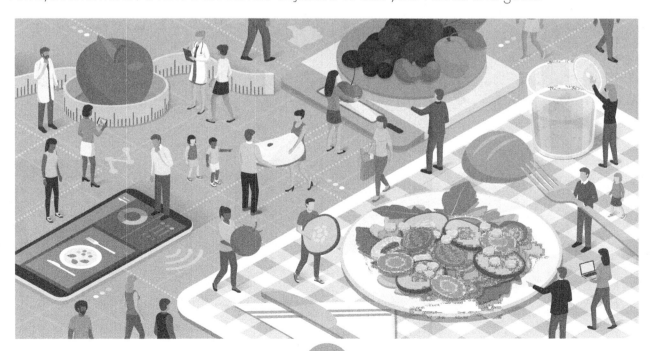

Keto Symptoms

The body may need a bit of time to adapt to using fat as its main energy source, especially if your body has been running on carbohydrates as its main energy source for a long period of time. Sometimes there are some symptoms involved during this period of adaptation. These symptoms are called the "keto flu," an experienced set of side-effects associated with carbohydrate withdrawal. Some of these symptoms include: headaches, dizziness, cramps/sore muscles, nausea, fatigue, irritability, mood swings, cravings, stomach pain/constipation, brain fog and insomnia. The "keto flu" symptoms usually disappear by themselves within a few days, as the body adapts. Here are a few tips to help you cure some of these symptoms faster if you experience the 'keto flu' symptoms. Drink a glass of water with a teaspoon of sea salt stirred into it at least once a day. You can also have bone broth as a tasty alternative with salt. In addition having electrolytes and B vitamins can help with this transition period. Make sure you also drink water when you are thirsty. Another tip is in the beginning stages take it easy with exercise and increase the intensity over a few weeks. Once you are over the "keto flu" symptoms you will soon be reaping all the benefits of your body being in a state of ketosis.

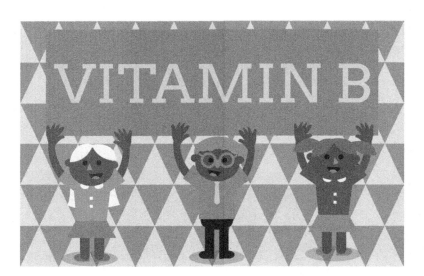
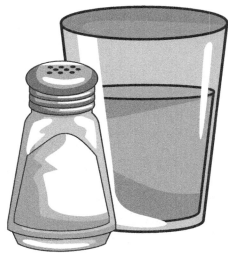
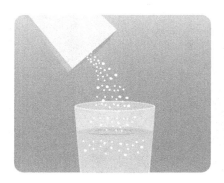
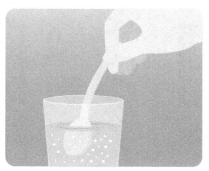
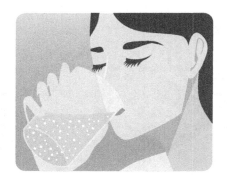

Intermittent Fasting on a Keto Diet

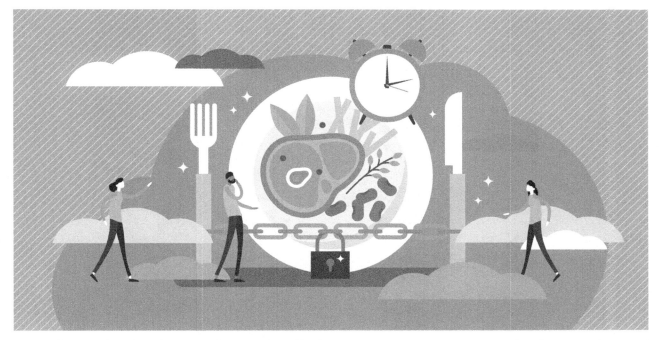

Intermittent fasting is actually a critically important step one can take for accelerated weight loss and maintaining ketosis.

One can take the keto diet to the next level by implementing a scheduled eating pattern called intermittent fasting. The benefit of intermittent fasting is that it shifts the body more readily into ketosis and one will discover that going longer periods of time without eating will be no problem since the body will be feeding off stored fat. Though one may be on the keto diet primarily to return to an ideal weight, the greatest benefit of intermittent fasting is the increase in health and resistance to diseases. Many studies show that this type of fasting while on the keto diet, helps the body's ability to ward off diseases such as cancer, Alzheimer's, Diabetes and more will be strengthened as a result.

Here's how this works: One already goes on an intermittent fast, every night. One is asleep for seven hours or so during which time one eats no food, right? That is many hours of fasting already. One can take it up a notch. Instead of eating three meals per day, possibly even with snacking in between, one would first start by cutting out any snacks between meals. Then start skipping breakfast to extend the fasting period. This can be done on a gradient by slowly having breakfast later and later in the day until you are eating "breakfast" at lunchtime. The goal for intermittent fasting would be to only eat two meals per day within a six hour window. One meal around lunchtime and the last one at dinner time. That would give one a daily fasting period of up to eighteen hours. One cup of coffee or tea first thing in the morning is fine if needed.

One will soon discover that eating on this schedule is very simple. One will feel energetic, mentally sharp and surprisingly one won't even feel hungry during these fasting periods. Many people are also amazed at the weight loss boost one gets from intermittent fasting.

Chapter 7

Let the Keto Journey Begin

You have finally decided. Take the leap into a healthier, more fit and you knowing that science has proven the workability of your decision. Your journey will lead you on a path of not only better health, but also towards a strong mental state. So, let's get the ball rolling and make it happen!

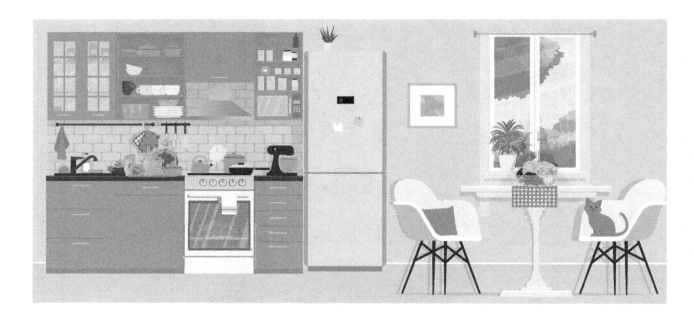

Time to Clean Out the Pantry

That pantry in your kitchen has had years of being restocked with sugars and carbs. It needs a major spring cleaning. Take all these items and put them in a box and then walk down to a homeless shelter and donate them. In addition to putting these things out of your way, you just performed a random act of kindness. Involve your family, it helps if you all are in it together. If they don't want to, it's okay. Your results will show them the way.

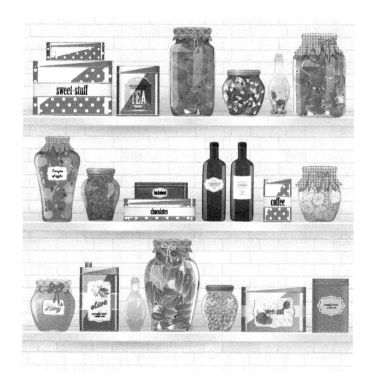

Weigh Yourself

You need to know where you are so you can measure how far you have come. You may notice a little gain initially, but don't lose hope. Remember it's a process and it will get better as your body gets used to it. You don't have to weigh yourself every day and stress over when the scale doesn't go in the right direction. Losing weight on the Keto Diet is not always linear. It can happen in fits and starts. Just hang in there and soon enough you will enjoy the results.

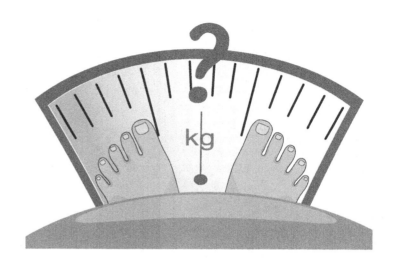

Get Smart With Substitutes

Remember those cheesecakes that you loved so much? Or those mashed potatoes which were on your plate every time? Yes, you won't be eating them on a Keto Diet, but you will be able to find low-carb substitutes.

There are always recipes that will provide you with a similar dish without the negative side effects. Try to swap a carb-rich ingredient of your favorite food with something more keto-friendly. A lettuce wrap is an excellent substitute for a carb-laden taco shell. Grated cauliflower may be the answer to your mashed potato cravings. Ever try the 'zoodles'? Its noodles made from zucchini. We are all born creative, let's use a bit of it when looking at the things we eat.

We at Ketoveo have published a number of cookbooks containing literally thousands of recipes in order to to make it easy for you to choose and make healthy, tasty and fulfilling keto-friendly breakfasts, lunches, dinners and desserts. Go to Ketoveo.com to see all of our various cookbook choices.

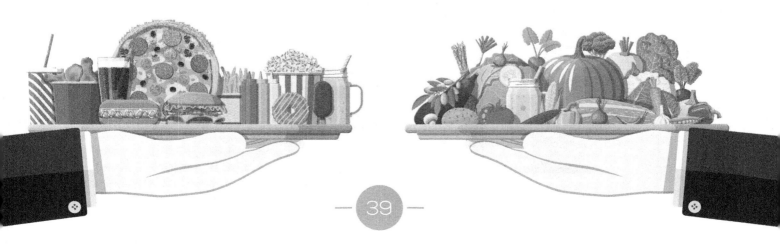

Condiments are Not Your Friend

If you ever thought that ketchup is healthy, think again. Ketchup is filled with sugar. Read the label of your everyday condiments and you will be surprised at what you find. Keep your guard up against salad dressings at restaurants. It's better to ask what they are made of instead of eating and going on a sugar trip

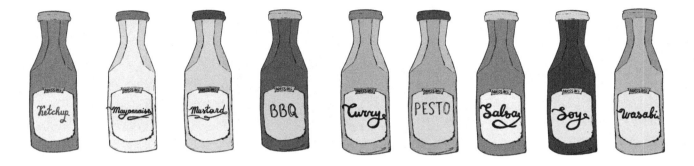

Watch Your Ketones

Keep an eye on your ketone levels. It is an important step to know what is happening inside of your liver with those ketones. It is a simple urine test, using keto-strips which we have available also on our website Ketoveo.com. Do it first thing in the morning to get the most accurate read.

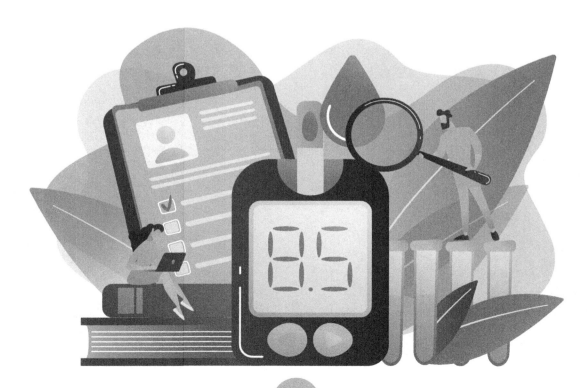

What About Eating Out?

You might be thinking: a Keto Diet would mean an end to eating out, right? Absolutely not! You merely have to choose your foods wisely, always keeping in mind what your goals are in terms of carbs, proteins, and fats. There are plenty of things available on most good restaurant menus to choose from so you need not worry overmuch. This will keep you on track and allow you to still enjoy your favorite restaurants.

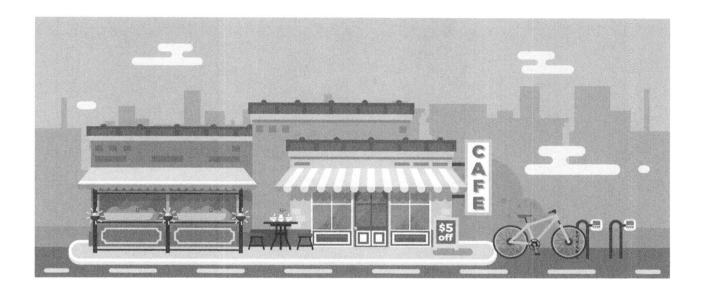

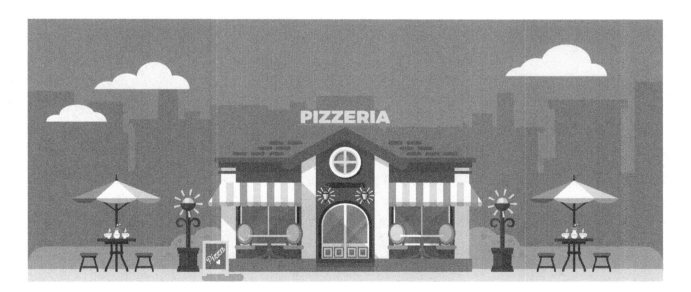

Get Your Protein & Exercise

A Keto Diet with plenty of protein will help your body build muscle as long as you include a healthy amount of exercise. Make exercise a part of your routine. Keep it simple. If you can't make it to the gym, get creative at home.

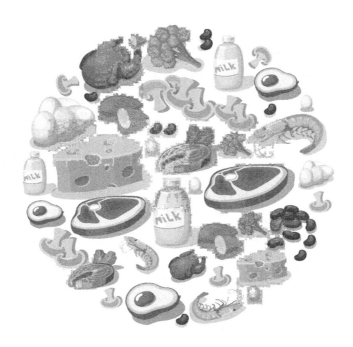

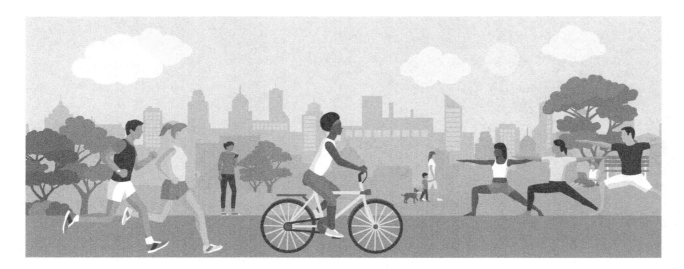

Endgame

In a few months, after having embraced the Keto lifestyle, you will look better, feel better, and you will be amazed at your surge in energy. You have made choices which have tested your willpower, but you have done it.

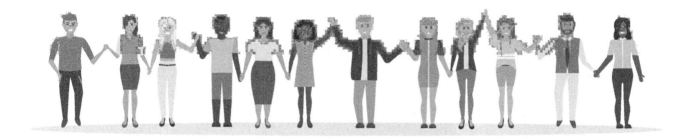

So what is next? Once you have lost those extra pounds or improved your health, you need to keep going. It is often said, 'It's easier to reach the top than it is to stay there." Do not stop, keep going, keep those carbs away and let your ketones do their job. It will enrich you and inspire others around you. You have come a long way, enjoy the journey, enjoy the process. Have a great Keto life.

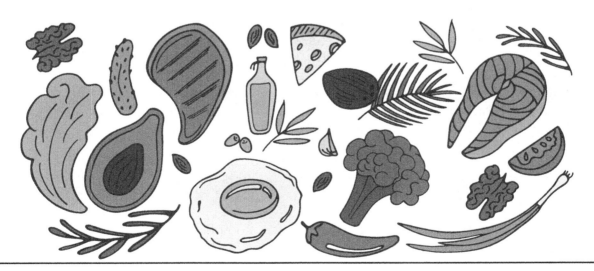

GLOSSARY

Alzheimer's Disease: A disease of the brain that causes people to slowly lose their memory and mental abilities.

Antioxidants: Substances produced by the body and found in foods which defend your body from damage caused by harmful forms of oxygen molecules called free-radicals.

Autism: A condition that begins in childhood that causes problems in forming relationships and in communicating with other people.

Calorie: A unit of food energy.

Carbohydrates: Any one of various substances in food (sugars, starches and fibers found in fruits, grains, vegetables and milk products) that are commonly used as fuel for your body to produce heat and energy.

Diabetes: A serious disease in which the body cannot properly control the amount of sugar in the blood because it does not produce enough insulin; a hormone produced by the pancreas.

Diet: A controlled regimen of the type and amount of food that a person eats for a certain reason, such as to improve health or to lose weight.

Fat: Fat is a source of fuel; for energy to run the body, and for process to maintain health. When fat is produced by the body that is not immediately needed, the body stores the fat for future use and energy.

Fatty acids: These are very high-energy fuels. Fatty acids are the building blocks of the fat in our bodies. When the body needs to use the fat as a fuel, it breaks the fat back down into fatty-acids which can then be absorbed into the blood.

Free radicals: Molecules that are highly reactive forms of oxygen which can damage cells. It is believed that having too many free radicals in the body accelerates the progression of cancer, cardiovascular disease, and age-related diseases.

Glucose: Simple sugars the body produces from carbohydrates which the body uses as a fuel. Glucose is preferred by the body as it can use this quicker and easier than fat. When the body produces more glucose than it needs, it converts it to Glycogen and stores it.

Glycogen: A compound made up of many glucose molecules which are then stored in muscles and the liver for later use as a fuel. The body can only store a limited amount of glycogen so when it produces too much, the body converts it to fat. All the glycogen stored in the body will be burned up in one day of fasting.

Hayflick limit: When a cell divides, it makes new cells. A cell divides again and again until it reaches the Hayflick limit, usually about fifty and seventy divisions, and then the cell dies.

IGF-1: This is an abbreviation that stands for Insulin-like Growth Factor #1. IGF-1 is a protein made by the liver that stimulates the growth of many types of cells and is similar to insulin. Intermittent fasting on the Keto Diet controls the production of IGF-1.

Inflammation: The body's reaction to injury or infection. The five common signs of inflammation are heat, pain, redness, swelling, and loss of function in the area affected.

Insulin: A hormone that lowers the level of glucose in the blood. It is released into the blood when the glucose level goes up, such as after eating. Insulin helps glucose enter the body's cells, where it can be used for energy or stored for future use.

Ketogenic diet: A diet high in fat, low in carbohydrates (sugars) and an adequate amount of protein. The diet forces the body take fat and convert it to ketones which then become the fuel your body uses to power the body.

Ketosis: A normal metabolic process that takes place when the body does not have glucose to use as its source of energy. When a body is "in ketosis", it uses fat as its primary fuel.

Ketones: When the body breaks down fat into fatty acids, it then breaks down the fatty acids into ketones. Ketones are used by the mitochondria in the cell to become energy for the brain, heart and muscles.

Keto Flu: A collection of symptoms experienced by some people when they first start the keto diet. These symptoms, which can feel similar to the flu, are caused by the body adapting to a new diet consisting of very little carbohydrates.

Liver: A large organ of the body that produces bile and cleans the blood. The liver is one of the largest organs in the body. It has many important functions. It converts the nutrients from food into chemicals the body can use. It stores these substances and supplies cells with them when needed.

Medium-chain triglycerides (MCTs): Triglycerides are the major form of fat in the body. They come from the food we eat as well as from being made by the body. MCTs produce more ketones per unit of energy than normal dietary fats. They influence a feeling of fullness and prevent hunger pangs. Rich food sources of MCTs include coconut oil, palm kernel oil, and dairy products.

Mitochondria: These are tiny "organs" inside the cells which produce the energy the body needs to function. 70% of the energy produced by mitochondria are used by the brain. Cells contain from 1000 to 2500 mitochondria.

Omega-3: A type of fatty acid that lowers cholesterol in the blood, protects against late age-related eye disease and is good for your heart. It is found in salmon and other fish as well as in green leafy vegetables, and some nuts.

Omega-6: A type of fatty acid that lowers cholesterol and reduces the risk of heart disease. A body needs to have it but cannot produce it by itself. Omega-6 fatty acids come from many vegetable oils, nuts, beans, seeds and grains.

Oxidative stress: An imbalance between the production of free radicals and the ability of the body to defend against their harmful effects. Oxidative stress can destroy cells and increase the risk of cancer.

Pancreas: A large gland of the body that is behind the stomach and that produces insulin and other substances that help the body digest food.

Protein: A nutrient found in foods such as meat, milk, eggs, and beans that is a necessary part of the diet and is essential for normal cell structure, muscle and function.

Sebum: Is an oily substance produced by glands in your skin which act as a lubricant for the hair and skin. It also provides some protection against bacteria and helps preserve the flexibility of the hair.

Starch: A carbohydrate that is found in certain foods, such as bread, rice, and potatoes. The body turns starch into glucose for use as a fuel.

Sugar: A sweet substance especially from the plants sugar cane and sugar beet, used to make food and drinks sweet. The body turns sugar into glucose for use as a fuel.

Made in the USA
Coppell, TX
07 July 2020